IMMUNOLOGY AND IMMUNE SYSTEM DISORDERS

LIVING A CELIAC LIFE

IMMUNOLOGY AND IMMUNE SYSTEM DISORDERS

Additional books in this series can be found on Nova's website under the Series tab.

Additional e-books in this series can be found on Nova's website under the e-book tab.

IMMUNOLOGY AND IMMUNE SYSTEM DISORDERS

LIVING A CELIAC LIFE

TIZIANA BEATO
CAROLINA CIACCI
AND
MONICA SINISCALCHI

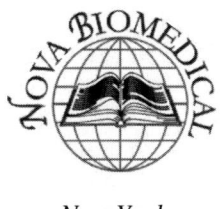

New York

Copyright © 2014 by Nova Science Publishers, Inc.

All rights reserved. No part of this book may be reproduced, stored in a retrieval system or transmitted in any form or by any means: electronic, electrostatic, magnetic, tape, mechanical photocopying, recording or otherwise without the written permission of the Publisher.

For permission to use material from this book please contact us:
Telephone 631-231-7269; Fax 631-231-8175
Web Site: http://www.novapublishers.com

NOTICE TO THE READER

The Publisher has taken reasonable care in the preparation of this book, but makes no expressed or implied warranty of any kind and assumes no responsibility for any errors or omissions. No liability is assumed for incidental or consequential damages in connection with or arising out of information contained in this book. The Publisher shall not be liable for any special, consequential, or exemplary damages resulting, in whole or in part, from the readers' use of, or reliance upon, this material. Any parts of this book based on government reports are so indicated and copyright is claimed for those parts to the extent applicable to compilations of such works.

Independent verification should be sought for any data, advice or recommendations contained in this book. In addition, no responsibility is assumed by the publisher for any injury and/or damage to persons or property arising from any methods, products, instructions, ideas or otherwise contained in this publication.

This publication is designed to provide accurate and authoritative information with regard to the subject matter covered herein. It is sold with the clear understanding that the Publisher is not engaged in rendering legal or any other professional services. If legal or any other expert assistance is required, the services of a competent person should be sought. FROM A DECLARATION OF PARTICIPANTS JOINTLY ADOPTED BY A COMMITTEE OF THE AMERICAN BAR ASSOCIATION AND A COMMITTEE OF PUBLISHERS.

Additional color graphics may be available in the e-book version of this book.

Library of Congress Cataloging-in-Publication Data

ISBN: 978-1-62948-803-5

Library of Congress Control Number: 2014930665

Published by Nova Science Publishers, Inc. † New York

Contents

Foreword		vii
Acknowledgments		ix
Chapter I	Viola	1
Chapter II	Annamaria	3
Chapter III	Giulia	5
Chapter IV	Viola	7
Chapter V	Annamaria	9
Chapter VI	Giulia	13
Chapter VII	Annamaria and Giulia	15
Chapter VIII	Viola and Mamma	17
Chapter IX	Annamaria and the Chef	19
Chapter X	Annamaria	21
Chapter XI	Viola	23
Chapter XII	Annamaria	25
Chapter XIII	Viola	27
Chapter XIV	Annamaria	29
Chapter XV	Giulia	31
Chapter XVI	Annamaria	33

Chapter XVII	Mamma	35
Chapter XVIII	Viola	39
Chapter XIX	Annamaria	43
Chapter XX	Mamma	47
Chapter XXI	Viola	49
Chapter XXII	Readers' Guide	51
Chapter XXIII	Medical Notes	53
Authors' Contact Information		69
Index		71

Foreword

Three women who meet downtown around a coffee table on a windy day that moves the menus and ideas equally. Their jobs, which so often force them to discuss the way they talk about the unease, about the disease, without being boring. The idea: a book, such as a novel, that would appeal to everyone and help them to understand what living a celiac life means.

The people and the facts in this book are real. Thus the experiences, thoughts and words we relate come directly from the stories of those who live with gluten intolerance. Annamaria stands for the hundred doctors in the world who treat patients with celiac disease or other food intolerances every day; Giulia represents the psychologists who help them overcome the changes in lifestyle the disease demands; Viola represents all the celiac patients who suddenly see their life change, luckily for the better.

We enjoyed describing a world that we know well and living in that world, for once in our lives, through this novel, although as close to reality as possible.

We dedicate this book to all of the patients whose personal experiences we have summoned up hereby; they have preoccupied our lives both professionally and emotionally.

Acknowledgments

The authors are grateful to Prof. Laura Caliendo for her translation. Her wise advice enriched and improved their work, allowing them to share their experience with a larger part of the celiac and non-celiac celiac world. They are also thankful to Daniel V. Di Giacomo for his friendly support and suggestions.

Chapter I

Viola

My eyes are still tired.

My eyelids always open up like an alarm to warn that my stop is the next one. At this early hour everyone sleeps on the subway, bags over their shoulders. I let the brisk halts lull me as I look at these human beings going to work, and who will surely phone someone the moment they get off the train.

I will phone no one. I am a colourless researcher at the Contemporary Arts Institute though, actually, I do not do any research, I catalogue. I catalogue catalogues.

On the train my thoughts run on the rails and, in spite of the hundreds of people around me, in my heart I know that I'm the only one to blame if all my relationships come to an end. It always happens like that: as soon as I feel that my emotional and romantic self becomes involved, I just start to drag down meetings, try not to answer calls and use unthinkable excuses to turn down dates.

Then I just disappear, like summer holiday memories that leave no trace. I avoid human beings and I perceive them as nails tearing and biting into my flesh. The subway is faster than my logic and I must put my thoughts aside.

Piazza Mazzini. A two-hundred-metre run to the usual coffee shop for my barley coffee and then straight to work.

A routine that's hard to break, like when you are at a roulette table, short on money yet go on gambling anyway, kidding yourself the ball will stop on your number. Yet it never does.

At the coffee shop words taste of coffee and chocolate.

A few people are discussing a film, the same old story where he leaves his wife for the cold blonde, the foreigner with the shapely long legs. They flee to Amsterdam, open a coffee shop and have three children.

Unnoticed I listen to them, well, I did like that film.

After all it is daring of him to change his life in one breath, to reverse the spinning of his own world and to counter the gravity which keeps us glued to the sofa after dinner watching the film we love best.

I too ran away from home. I didn't truly mean to run away, I'd say it was more like a long holiday to find myself again, or better still, to understand my thoughtful, and at times, immature self. Six years ago I started to pack books, CDs and jewellery boxes. My mother thought I was simply training for evacuation even though our house is in a quiet and peaceful village. She didn't ask the reason for my leaving, as it were just a long holiday; too strong her love, too exaggerated my devotion to her.

"Good morning Viola!" Marilù the secretary says and her look hits me in the face like a punch, as she checks the clock behind me.

The Institute has lost five minutes of my neurons. At the back of the small room, like dried flowers to throw away, the catalogues are waiting for my obsessive attention to be ordered according to title, author, publisher, number of pages, publication year, colour, thickness and amount of dust in microns that I calculate by the number of sneezes they bring on.

Catalogues are not human beings thus I can simply deal with them. Nevertheless, since I started cataloguing, I have discovered that I have a dust allergy and since I've been working here, my belly groans, roars, murmurs, twists and tightens.

I'm using up the tiles going to and fro between the toilet and the catalogues. Irritable bowel syndrome, the doctor stated. Whatever it is, it makes my life impossible.

I find myself face to face with the calm and silent solitude of every single day of work.

Like a day in a prison with no bars, a videogame with the same scenery, I play, but the background never changes.

Chapter II

Annamaria

The metro in Rome stinks. I can't help thinking that at this very moment billions of germs are dancing on the train, an extemporaneous 'macumba' for a chosen person who will have a swollen face and a hacking, hollow cough in a few weeks. Too many, too many people we are and the narrow and unfit spaces we populate result in an exchange of viruses, bacteria, dead cells that fall on my shoulders and mix with the hairspray.

I watch the pilgrims in this filthy car, are they resigned or calm, I wonder. As I always travel by car and don't even notice those next to me in the traffic I notice that the subway, instead, forces you to observe, to anthropologically analyse.

This morning my car didn't want to leave the garage like a nut that doesn't want to leave its shell. Thanks to my car's will I have to socialise with other people's germs.

I'm pushed to Piazza Mazzini.

My hospital is on Piazza Mazzini. Well, not that I own a hospital. Anyway, I've been spending more time there than at home. When you have been working in a place for more than twenty years it becomes your place. When you work shifts or fight for yourself and your colleagues and especially when you know that at least thirty patients are waiting outside your room hanging on your every word as on an oracle's, then you are the hospital's and the hospital is yours. They greet me at the entrance and still they are only voices; as soon as I enter this healing temple, I become alienated, all my thoughts focus on what I have to do, what to say and the ones I have to see. I forget I'm hungry or in need of the bathroom, I just feel I have to serve my patients and the hospital.

A. Mancini, M.D. Room 416. Gastroenterology Unit. That's me. My whole life is on that doorplate. Nevertheless a plaque could not relate the sacrifices, the mistakes, the choices, my baby's diapers, the out of town excursions with the family, my husband's surprise birthday parties - mostly unsuccessful - the years abroad, the plane that didn't take off and the increasing anxiety before sleeping. It's too much to put on a plaque. I wear the white coat. I leave it loose since I do nothing risky or dangerous, besides I choose my outfits carefully. I inherited this trait from my mother who never wore house dresses and slippers and thus didn't want her daughters to either. And so I float between being a doctor and a vain woman.

Chapter III

Giulia

They are laughing. I'm smiling too as I look at the two boys sitting opposite me, they are plotting, they look at me and laugh. I want to share. We start a game of looks, I try to understand what they are pointing at, what fun lies there, but there are too many people around. After all, it is difficult to interpret something in a subway. From my seat near the window I can only see skirts and jeans, I barely see faces, and I rely on the eyes of the boys who surely have something better to look at above my head. Still they are nice, young and it's good that they laugh, I like them. I think that to start a day with a laugh does a lot of good to your blood, brain and soul. I always want to see the glass as half full and I try to turn a negative factor into a positive one, just viewing it from an unusual, different perspective. Professional bias, I admit it. My job is to help people face the diseases of the soul, psychological distortions and behavioural disorders.

The subway certainly proves to be a very good place for people who do my job. I keep looking at the boys, but they don't want me in their game, they talk using slang, a sort of code; I'm clearly the one who can't get it and there are no interpreters around, thus I give up and open my mobile.

A plump man approaches me, he wears turtle framed glasses, has a repentant teddy-bear face and makes his way along the aisle pushing people with a lot of 'sorry,' 'please,' 'sorry,' 'just a moment,' 'please,' 'may I,' 'let me through.' Eventually he reaches me with a satisfied air as if to show that nothing can stop him and that he has made it all the way just for me. In a single breath, he says:

"Hello, Giulia lets get off together and have a coffee." "What about having lunch together?" "That's all right, don't worry!"

About the man: Giovanni, a social worker, 1.60 cm tall, mostly words and ham sandwiches, always on foot. He still lives with his mother and a cat.

About me: Giulia Castaldi, a psychotherapist whose name is now at the mercy of everyone on the train. I reply with a 'yes,' fearing that he could have an embolism if he carries on speaking this way. Piazza Mazzini station, not difficult to get off; Giovanni leads the way and I descend the stairs in triumph like The Snow Queen.

Chapter IV

Viola

    I'm biting my nails, they are tasteless, still, for a few moments they stave off my hunger and prevent me from strolling out for an ice-cream. The others are in the refreshment bar. A clattering of forks, glasses and cans, a wagging of jaws and the crumpling of plastic fills the air. A continuous hiss, a sort of snail that propels me forward, towards the forbidden fruit, a heaven of mini pizzas, rice salads and fizzy drinks. I'm hungry, yet I eat nothing. A kind of exhaustion has been affecting my muscles and thoughts for days and so the catalogues lay on the shelves. A young Bacchus by Caravaggio looks at me from a cover. I smile at him, recognising myself in his gloomy look. I'm not turning purplish like the young Bacchus! I run to the mirror and place the catalogue near my face for comparison. My skin is fair and, on the contrary, it is he who is much too wasted.

    You are the sick one, damned Bacchus!

    I'm only feeling sick, you can't say I am, at least not until deemed so by a specialist. The damp patches on the mirror make my face appear patched. I can see myself at waist length, a 156 cm woman, all knowledge and bad humour. My high cheek bones ready to confront the world. Marilù notices my thinness and every morning she says, "How can you be so in shape, Miss Viola?" May it be love that keeps you off your food?" Love? This word puzzles me. To me love is like chasing a hare that, once caught, you set free, feeling guilty. What excites me is the hunt, the placing of the snares and traps. The best part of love is waiting for the catch. I need some fresh early November air.

    I head for the square where you can find a Neverland for ladies. Rare pieces of plastic bijouterie, shirts, belts, impossible scarves that you buy out of excitement because of their bargain price, then once at home, when the enchantment is over, you realise you will never wear them, not even for the housework. Since I have been away from my mother I have devotedly applied myself to glamour shopping, to colours, materials and accessories. It is a kind of daily carnival that lets me pretend to be anybody else, but me. I don't like Viola. I feel angry with myself, I could be shrewd and ironic, I know I could easily be in one of those television shows where you need an above average general knowledge to win. I think people don't like my true nature, fear me and set me apart. I guess human beings trust those people more who prove they are tender by being calm, shy and reverential, the ones who, thanks to their weaknesses, produce affection and a sort of natural fondness from the very first moment.

The boutique on the corner of the sidewalk is a private club for women, we all meet there during our lunch break. Then we exchange advice, suggest the right earrings or a trendy skirt and become friends. I decide to buy something; I wander like a sly cat among the shelves looking for a detail, a colour, an object waiting only for me. As I come out of the changing room with a yellow shirt on, a very tall chick stares at me shaking her head.

"Doesn't suit me?"

"It does nooot". You're very pale and this acid yellow clashes with your blue eyes. Have a look over there, there is a green t-shirt that will suit you. Better still, I'll fetch it. Is it an S or an M?" I hesitate, then say "M".

I look at her going up and down among the odalisques of this fashion harem. It's as if she is walking down the red carpet in Hollywood and, calm and smiling, comes back with her 'Oscar' shirt. "C'mon, try it on. I'll wait here." Quickly, as if in a sort of trance, I pull off my shirt, put on the green t-shirt, tidy up my hair and look at myself in her wide hazel eyes. "That's it! Take it. It suits you perfectly". I find myself in the queue at the cash desk, gripping in my hand the only garment worth buying, my green t-shirt, size M. I walk with a haughty air, clutching my trophy.

Chapter V

Annamaria

A mother comes in with a plump girl with an acne afflicted teenage face. It is the mother who takes the seat, speaks and looks at the photos on my desk. I welcome her with a smile as large as all my studies, seminars and meetings. I let her vent. I reckon that the lady needs to protest, to spit words out on her daughter, on me. I'm used to telling myself that a doctor needs a psychological diagnosis before a biophysical one so I pay attention. The mother tells me the girl has bouts of nausea before eating and that every morning she checks her weight, bursting into tears if the scales say three hundred grams more than usual. Some words get lost in the room. I turn to the girl who suddenly feels like the only protagonist of the day. She stares at me and starts to list more than fifty disorders, which are clearly too many even to a gastroenterologist. My sense of duty would normally demand the ordering of the usual routine tests, a scan and blood tests. My sixth sense however, which is always present, like my glasses, that I still never find, informs me that again I'm facing an insane family dynamic in which a girl wishing for a show girl body, clearly has food behavioural disorders but not a food intolerance.

I think of my daughter, of the freedom I gave her, partly due to my long absences due to work.

Every day I relate to mothers and daughters as patients who depend on each other, whereas my daughter even at thirteen, could cook a decent meal for herself and her father. I'd even say she is a better cook than I am now. I suggest to the mother-daughter pair that they see a psychologist first. Then we'll see, assuring them there are no signs suggesting an obscure food intolerance.

I've been focusing my interest on food intolerance and celiac celiac disease for years. Celiac Celiac disease is very interesting. I hate to call it a disease. I wouldn't call it a disease but a fact, like having dark eyes or fair hair. You are celiac and that's that. Every day I discuss it with patients, with colleagues in seminars, with my friends at home and still feel every time as if it were the first time, not only because the research is moving so quickly, but also because of the passion I put into it. I know a lot about celiac disease, I have studied it, done research in labs and crunched thousands of numbers, compiled thousands of tables and seen thousands of patients. I've lived more with celiac disease than with my family.

I haven't got numbers, medical records and procedures in front of me, but real names and surnames, smiles, gazes, readers and movie-makers, housewives, students and teachers.

I put my thoughts aside and welcome the next patient, a young lad with a thin fair beard, very thin and glaring eyes rich with ambition and future projects. He is young and, uninvited, takes his seat boldly in front of me. I raise a welcoming smile. The young lad feels embarrassed, he has to tell me about himself. First he tells me he is an artist, better still he draws and makes sketches for theatres, several customers, and he shows me some comic strips as well. He is enthusiastic about his work and I reckon that he starts by speaking about it because that is what the disease stopped.

He no longer has the strength to draw. He can't sleep at night and feels tired during the day. As he goes on talking, I look at his works; his stroke is like a wave, a slash of water across the face. They are amusing but show a studied technique and commitment.

He is a sad artist but a sad artist produces nothing. Sadness stops everything whereas happiness gives life even to unthinkable ideas. He feels tired, useless, spends a lot of time on a sofa never feeling like going out, not even with his girlfriend. He has no bowel symptoms. He has come to me after hearing on TV that some people who always feel tired may suffer from a food intolerance; so he decided to be tested for celiac disease. Actually he is a coeliac, a depressed and bewildered person. Only one word comes to my mind: time. Let his new diet heal his bowel and give him new energy. I say it vigorously as if to rouse him from an emotional sleep, not his own. I'll see him soon, 'goodbye.' He leaves an unfinished sketch behind.

I think, 'it will be finished.'

I'm tired and nervous. I leave the hospital and head for a small shop where spending money seems natural, so various are the brightly coloured and sweet smelling objects. I enjoy trying things on and, to an even greater degree, finding, among the customers, a 'babe' to give my dispassionate advice to.

Today the babe to undress and dress anew is a pretty little woman about thirty with lovely sad wide eyes. She emerges from the dressing room like an alien, wearing a yellow shirt that clashes with her pale face and eyes. I choose a light green t-shirt that will make her day. Here she is: a large sized Barbie in a new dress. She thanks me. I smile at her. I seldom buy something but I make decisions for the lonely and desperate women who can't make up their minds, standing in front of a pair of silver earrings worth €5. It's so easy, 'you will never wear them, but buy them all the same, because a touch of originality is worth €5.

Chapter VI

Giulia

He's crying and I've already handed him three tissues. His wife, fed up with him being a sick person with no diagnosis, left him for a handsome boy with a supersonic twin-turbo. Although I know he is crying, I can't help thinking that she is on the coast having fun with her porcelain-smile boy toy. I stare at him as he finally stops crying.

He is the last patient of the day. Not that all of them cry, still they all need a better life; to learn how to manage with their emotions. The abandoned husband calms down, talks about his bowels, shows me the list of the food he cannot tolerate it's a long list. While I'm reading it, he says that when he is emotionally unbalanced it gets even worse. It used to happen before exams when he was a boy and is happening again now that he is facing a separation. His doctor suggested that he see a psychologist to help him overcome the emotional trauma that is upsetting his bowels. I listen to him, I would hug him, but luckily I can't: professional ethics. Thus I grip my ever-present silk scarf, which is a means to restrain my own repressed love. Anyway I simply can't analyse myself while analysing him. I hope something will change in his life after seeing me. To me it's important to be ready to change.

My favourite hobby? Changing.

For instance: I play checkers with my furniture. Moving is reinventing; I move every three months though I live in the same flat. I'm certain, therefore, that changing is up to us and doesn't depend on external conditions. My beloved furniture is often my ally for turning an exasperating afternoon into a wonderful theatre, as I am the one to plan and make new sceneries according to the play I am going to live. The last patient leaves. I take a long walk which helps to loosen up my muscles and thoughts. During the analyses (shall we call them that?) I drift away from the earth with my feet in the air, I turn my thoughts off and I open the 'think box' where the patients, unknowingly, throw their words and tears, insults, anxieties and unrepeatable fancies.

I welcome them to this 'think box' that only the patient and I can use, discard the useless words, or the ones that are fit for a new change; a new chapter in their lives.

Of course, the discarded words are pieces of a puzzle, which, rearranged in the right order, make a new picture; my office is a permanent art exhibition.

Walking allows me to come back to myself, to the bills to pay, to the now rancid sauce left in the fridge a week ago. I walk around the square at least three times; I am curious, that is my nature. I think that it's beautiful to take step after step along the same stretch of street over and over, watching people in discussion, gesticulating with lips and wide eyes; and then to pass again and watch how they have changed their attitude over the course of a few minutes or that they have gone. The best spot is inside Divina's which is a sort of island of low cost luxury. I look at the customers; they are like queen bees in a hive, in a sea of honey. They exchange a pair of jeans with two sweaters back from the 70s; they push to grab a wicker basket, a cherry lipstick. They make a kind of 'female' friendship that can outface any world war; they are all for one, one for all.

Two bees in the hive exchange a t-shirt for a shirt and I sense that one is the leader and the other the fashion victim. I reckon the leader, Dc. Mancini, through her determination and self-confidence could make you change your mind in a split second. Her favourite hobby is buying everything online, from Chinese Christmas gifts to Wedgewood cups on e-bay. In other words, she is a real shopaholic, not just a pack rat however, that buys objects she will never use or means to lock away in a chest. I focus on everything in this square. It has never changed to me or I may not have noticed it. Once I was coming back from a party at night, the square was beautiful, silent and understated, the stars in the sky with the moon reflected in the mullioned glass windows of the bell tower. I was fifteen at the time and had just experienced my first kiss. The square was never again to seem so beautiful.

Chapter VII

Annamaria and Giulia

Coffee machine, sugarless coffee, both witness to a five-minute break between two appointments. It is the meeting point of the ward where patients, doctors and nurses exchange a few words, opinions and criticism. The machine proves to be a sort of automatic confessional, distributing thoughts at only 50 cents a pop.

"Sugar, sweetener?" I know Annamaria will answer, "No," she doesn't trust sweeteners; still, I want to try to make her change her mind.

"No! Thanks, Giulia, better bitter-tasting than poisoned." Annamaria says with a smile in her eyes rather than on her lips.

"I saw you at Divina's, what have you been up to this time?" I say, smiling.

I have known her for years and I enjoy listening to her contemporary, personal theories on the life-styles and socio-anthropologic trends of our technologically advanced planet that foists improvements and changes on us every fifteen minutes.

"Oh I couldn't keep silent, this time!" I say. That small, pale woman and her acid yellow shirt; a terrible match that naturally deters the other sex. No doubt, a light green t-shirt be much better in bringing out the poor wretch's eyes, allowing for a quick reintegration into society. Green stands for stability, strength and constancy. Moreover, it means self-confidence. Green is the colour of woods, nature and life itself."

She turns serious and her theories on fashion convince me; she seems taller than she is; there is a light in her eyes and an immediate satisfaction that would give a thrill to even the highest member of the International School for Effective

Communication. While I am finishing my coffee Annamaria cuts off our brief conversation and stares at the passers-by in the street.

I can't follow her gaze. There are moments when each of us gets lost behind a glass and seem to be looking out but are actually looking into the far distance, beyond the buildings around us.

Our personal thoughts do not follow us into the hospital; we keep them in the car, at home or in a notepad. Therefore, unaware, we take a break to get lost beyond a glass window.

I don't remember how long it has been since I last heard from my sister or visited my friend in Tuscany and I can't say why my feet are stuck here on the road stretching between my house and the hospital.

Deep in my thoughts, I watch Annamaria. I know what moments like this mean as I often live them myself. I understand how difficult it is being in one place when you would like to be somewhere else. Moreover, there are moments when you wish to be alone as if loneliness would make everything clearer, more true. Beyond the glass there is a walk through skyscrapers; there is a cup of tea.

Chapter VIII

Viola and Mamma

"Mummyy? Mummyyyy!"

There are only four rooms a bathroom and a balcony among them, and only two windows yet, every time I come to see her, it is a treasure hunt. Here she is… in the bathroom, busy ordering her personal soap-bar collection; souvenirs from the travels my dad, relatives, neighbours and I have been on. Useless brightly coloured shrivelled bars collected in hotels, villages and motels around the world.

What shall I bring you from Mexico? A soap-bar.

If she had been there she wouldn't have been interested in the view, in the typical food or in the precious magnets; to her a soap-bar is the most intimate object; the true product of a journey. She can even tell the quality of hotels and places by the soap-bar's wrapping or the logo impressed on the paper, its shape and scent. More than a hundred travels collected in a basket on the washing machine. She dusts them off, smells them (even if many of them have lost their scent and colour) and reorganises them.

My mother collects everything.

She collects the neighbours' complaints, my fears, the odd and boring days, our relatives' wishes, gossip and outbursts. She gathers together, in her life, the stories and the facts of many others.

"Viola!" she has seen me.

I am between the doorjamb and the tub and she is on a stool holding her soap jewels.

"Is something wrong? To what do I owe your visit?" She stands up and raises her left eyebrow. Although she is sixty-five, to me, she is the same mother as when I was eight.

I know that inquisitive look but even today I wonder how she uncovers everything concerning my life simply by the way I breathe; the way I call on the intercom before going up; my way of moving into the room or sitting at the table. She knows what upsets me, however, she enjoys challenging herself and her eighth sense (she has gone far beyond the sixth), testing the telepathy between us.

The questioning begins.

"How are you doing? Is work all right? 'When will you meet someone who will become your fiancee? Have you got enough money? Are you eating properly? You are so pale, so weird, so..."

I do not answer. I follow her and she washes her hands, dries them quickly and draws near to her command post: the stove.

Food to defrost, fry, salt, dress and bake. She is the queen in these three square metres of a kingdom and will never abdicate. I open the fridge: ham and cheese; she prepares a sandwich. I sit down and start eating in silence. I show her my love; that I appreciate her love with every bite.

She sits down opposite me quietly.

"Mummy, I feel wretched. I've been feeling tired for days. I don't know; I guess I have a bowel infection. You know my gut is my weak point. I can't concentrate at work and I don't feel like doing anything."

"It may be the stress," she says. "If you stayed at home, you would be better. Yesterday I cooked a very good apple pie. Lentil soup today and, if you stay for lunch, we'll have cutlet and fries!"

I look at her. I think of the cutlet and I feel upset. "Mummy I can't explain my general malaise."

"Go and see a doctor and have an examination; better today than tomorrow!"

"Better today than tomorrow," is her motto.

I imagine I'm hugging her, that she is reassuring and kissing me.

Chapter IX

Annamaria and the Chef

A dinner party at some friends' and I can't decline. Moreover, I want to go. I am glad to meet those people again who are so familiar to me; the people I have always known, who I feel close to and with whom I have shared films, holidays and my children's birthdays. Appointments are over and I rush home. I act like a teenager getting ready for a Saturday night out; I change my dress and put my hair in a ponytail. I go by taxi and am on time. All of my friends and my friends' friends are there. At dinner we discuss taxes, houses to buy or sell, separated friends and newborn grandchildren. I listen while staring at a young guy sitting opposite me, one of the host's friends. We both have the hint of a shy smile on our faces.

All of a sudden, as when you dive off a diving board, he starts talking.

"You are Dr Mancini, aren't you?"

"Yes, I am," I reply ...

"Well, have a look," He hands me a paper with dates and a meal for each (pizza, coke, pineapple, pasta with broccoli, baked chicken, strawberries). It is a list of his painful crises in the last months.

He plays it safe, "I'm under pressure," he says.

I'm bewildered. He knew I would be at the dinner and came to call for help.

He tells me that his younger brother died in an accident and now he realises that slowly all his irritable bowel symptoms are getting worse. He does not go out if he doesn't know where the bathroom is, he is spending a fortune on healthy food and he no longer drinks milk or eats pizza.

"It is the grief," they told him.

"Then I met Lucia eight months ago," he adds in a timid way.

Three months of living together: Lucia, a separated woman and her son with celiac disease. Out of curiosity and his partner's respect, he started to eat gluten-free food.

A miracle: the diarrhoea stops and the swollen belly is gone; in a few days the gluten-free diet makes him feel much better. In a couple of months, he goes to his doctor again. 'Could it be celiac disease?' It could, but, after being on a gluten-free diet for months, the blood test would say nothing because the antibodies would vanish. So the doctor suggests staying off the diet. Once again his belly becomes bloated and he does not feel well. He undergoes the tests, a blood sample is taken to check for antibodies and he even has a genetic test. They all are negative. It cannot be celiac disease. Yet he felt so much better. He tries gluten-free meals again and he feels much better.

I listen to him attentively and I look at him, he repeats that at present, he is gluten-free and with no symptoms but he still does not seem happy, why?

He tells me his secret: "I'm a chef, I do not want and I cannot have celiac disease. And since the tests show I don't have it, I'd like to ask you whether I'm nuts or I may have a different intolerance."

Another one, I think to myself, another one I can add to the clinical research on the non-celiac gluten sensitivity.

I speak slowly as one does when having to explain something important.

I tell him that, all over the world, some people without celiac disease think they are better off avoiding wheat and cereals.

"Might it be another element of wheat? Some sort of sugar we can find in cereals or vegetables and that we cannot digest? Might this sugar arrive at the colon undigested and thus feed bacteria that produce annoying gas pains?" "Well," I reply and talk about the theories, "There are no tests to show such intolerance. Patients identify it by themselves." My tablemate looks at me in bewilderment.

"How can I be sure it is not just an emotional factor? Can you prescribe a downer that allows me to eat everything with no fear?"

"Yeah," I say, "I could," while my thoughts go to Castaldi and to the emotional sphere.

I don't feel like eating anymore. We look at each other for a few seconds.

"Sorry for bothering you. Please, go on eating. It was me who cooked!"

Chapter X

Annamaria

I couldn't sleep. My thoughts kept going back to the chef and his intolerance; to his being distracted from life. When you don't feel well you get distracted; you lose sight of your job, of your passions, of love; unfortunately, you become concerned only with yourself because you feel ill. You can only focus on feeling better and going back to so called, 'normal life.'

Therefore I decide to go for a stroll. The freedom of wandering is beyond words because you can go to an unknown point for no reason, without pressure of limited time, with no one depending on you or to take care of.

I get to Divina's and I want to shop, to buy everything only to give this day a different sense. I realise I am the only one who takes things off the shelves without trying them on or looking at the price; spasmodically, I grasp items and throw them in the shopping bag like a starving tourist at a hotel self-service breakfast table. It's Friday, the last working day, the first relaxing day of the weekend. Divina's is as crowded as a theatre foyer on an opening night. I look around, hoping to see a friendly face, to find some female solidarity, but not one of the last minute fashion adventuresses can know the cause of my concern.

My eyes orbit the room like satellites. A noise startles me. A thud at my back, dummies and necklaces falling down. A sudden, sharp, dull noise I recognise.

Someone has fainted. Who is it?

The women are frantic; everyone gives her own opinion at a hundred words a second. The salesclerk lets out a hiss and then a cry of fright. "I am a doctor," I say. I don't like to intervene usually because I tend to think doctors can't actually do much in an emergency, out of the hospital and with no medical equipment, however I would feel guilty if I did not try.

I can see two feet jutting out of a mountain of woollen garments, shoes and shirts. I free the sleeping body. "Madam, madam!"

Customers and clerks get anxious and someone blows in her ear, some lift her arms and legs, and someone fetches some water. "Easy, easy. She is breathing; she has just fainted," I say and call for an ambulance. We go to the hospital; it is safer for her and it is safer for me.

Chapter XI

Viola

I don't know what happened. I feel light-headed. Just the fright, perhaps. I was at Divina's an hour ago because I had wanted to buy something nice for tomorrow night.

Now I am in an ambulance with the siren on. My arm hurts because they put a needle in the inside of my elbow; I am frightened. The woman that some time ago made me buy that green shirt at Divina's is in front of me. She pursues me: what does she want and who is she?

The woman is talking to me and I guess she is repeating the same things over and over. She is speaking in a low voice and is taking my pulse.

I fainted, we're going to the hospital and she is a doctor. She wants to know who I am. We dash through the hospital hall and into a room with many people and stretchers. I can hear the woman at my side call nurses and doctors by their names and give orders like a soldier.

My heart is thudding.

I'm thinking of my mother. I feel guilty; something different from what occurs in our ordinary lives has happened. A doctor arrives and I read the name on her badge: Dr Antonella Santini. She looks very young, with curly hair and small pearl earrings. She says she is a resident and has to ask me some questions. Once she starts nothing can stop her.

She makes me tell her what she needs to know. Then she asks me whether there is someone they can call, a relative or a friend. I don't know what to say and keep silent. Then, "No one, at the moment," I say, as I think that I will be all right and discharged. ER is always chaotic and if your ailment is nothing serious you will get IV therapy and that will be all. She examines the blood tests and I see a shadow in her eyes. She says I am anaemic and that I might have had some bleeding. They must keep me in and give me a transfusion. She calls the woman who was with me in the ambulance and who wears a white coat now. She too has a badge with a name: Dr A. Mancini

They are taking me to the x-ray department and afterwards to the ward.

The young doctor comes with me. While the stretcher speeds along the corridors, she asks about the symptoms from the previous weeks, about the diarrhoea.

Do I feel nauseous and tired? "Yes, I do. I have cramps as well."

The smell of the hospital annoys me and today it is especially strong. It goes straight from my nostrils to my brain and death and pain come to mind. Deep inside, I knew something was wrong and I knew I was becoming ill. I am afraid to leave my dear ones, to be unable to live a normal life or travel all over the world; to kiss a secret loved one, to buy a house or to finish the novel that lies on my night table.

I have seen people die; my father and my granny.

They will never know what they have left behind, the grief and the emptiness of the following days, or how much you miss them when you need their advice. I do not want to pass away without a real farewell.

Chapter XII

Annamaria

I had guessed that the girl who fainted was the one who had tried on that hideous shirt that highlighted her eye sockets at Divina's. Though, as an afterthought, she was pale; that's why yellow did not suit her. I go down quickly to the ER department. My heels echo down the stairwell. I ask about the blood count on the phone: "She is anaemic: the haemoglobin is 5.6."

Well, I have to arrange for admission and the scheduled routine. Luckily, Santini is in. She is almost perfect, like Mary Poppins, and updates me within a minute. The two of us get on the job while three nurses take her to the x-ray unit. So far, there is nothing more I can do, so I go up to my room and lock myself in. I can't do anything except wait for the next two hours. I start to surf the web to find exotic things to buy. I made a vow I wouldn't buy anything for seven days as I know that is my weak point. It is because of the money I spend but because of my thirst for buying things. I am reminded of what a psychologist told me some years ago, "This means you feel anxious." I can better understand other people's fears because they are mine as well. I don't want my anxiety to show through so I have learnt how to use it and turn it into my strong point. Giulia may be the only one who gets it. I like Giulia Castaldi because she is pragmatic. When she tells me about her patients I know she is eager to find a solution to their anxiety. Once, on the metro, I bumped into her along with a claustrophobic girl on a tour for therapeutic purposes. My Farmville farm on the PC screen is gorgeous; I plant flowers and vegetables and it resembles a sort of coloured chessboard when in bloom. I then take pictures and harvest everything. I began to play at the airport when I was waiting to board.

I hear people chatting in the corridor. I am tired, perhaps the never changing routine has taken its toll, and all my patients seem undistinguishable. Once it was different though; I remember Giulia telling me about 'burn-out' syndrome. When she did I didn't take it as referring to me, what if on the contrary, she were?

I search PubMed for information on the doctors' burn out.

Chapter XIII

Viola

"No! I will not do it."

"You are crazy." I've just realised what they want to do. I will not allow anyone to introduce a thin flexible instrument down my gullet and into my stomach. That is: I will not undergo a gastroscopy, as doctors call it. They look at me as if I am an alien; both the doctors and staff nurses (who wear uniforms of a different colour) are bewildered by my childish behaviour. When scared I revert to my childish behaviour and though I am aware of the interior transformation I can't control myself and feel ashamed afterwards. I do not want to undergo a gastroscopy simply because I'm scared.

"When I say no, I mean it, like right now. I will win."

My voice turns thin and tremulous; I clench my fists and strain my muscles. "You can tie me up; I still will not undergo a gastroscopy." The doctors try to explain the importance of this test; how painless and especially how necessary it is to make a diagnosis. A video camera in my stomach? No, thanks.

It's hard to convince me and by now the score is one-zero. They are losing their patience.

Although I do not feel well, with a pale face and cramp in my legs, the 'no' I insist on gives me strength; I feel invincible.

I see the doctors and Dr Santini hatching a new plan. They approach me and say they can understand me and my reaction, which is normal. However the point is that the gastroscopy is necessary. Now the medical firing squad executes plan B.

They decide I need help, some support, to face the test and what will follow afterwards.

A female doctor will take care of me it is decided; I guess she is, more than a doctor, a kind of guide for the scared. I gather their plan B is to ease the situation with the help of this hospital shaman who, with only the power of her mind, will get me to accept to be sedated, open my mouth, relax and allow that endoscope down into my stomach.

Chapter XIV

Annamaria

    It's still a 'no' and I'm certainly not happy to impose a gastroscopy. In addition, she is one of those patients who view the test as an assault, a useless imposition. How arrogant. They also get angry and angry at me. And I too get angry at them. I'm fed up with pounding away. You don't want to? Well, don't then. I know how my heart quickens at the stress of intubating a patient.

    The statistical data is that one out of every thousand patients bleeds, one will suffer a perforation and one out of every million dies. Who will that 'one' be? Will it be just you, the damned one of my fears?

    Moreover, what if the anaemia is caused by a bleeding ulcer? You are young, all right but you are not immune to the disease. I do not have the other test results yet, however, your face tells me it is celiac disease, not an ulcer. The white, thin almost translucent skin says it and the blue lines under your eyes; the high cheekbones in a thin, long face and the brittle hair say it. You are slim and suffer gastrointestinal symptoms. In a bet I'd be the winner. The head nurse says I have developed a sixth sense for celiac disease.

    Let's play the game. You are new at the game as the main player whereas I've been playing it for years. You'll say 'no,' I'll say 'yes,' I'll scare you and then I'll comfort and reassure you, and in the end I'll get your consent.

    I hope Castaldi will soften you up. She has a good technique. She is sympathetic and warm but resolute as well. I like to see her contain the patients' anxiety. Containment, she calls it. She builds a dyke, a super dyke worthy of a National Geographic documentary. Perhaps now a mild anxiolytic would do the trick. Sometimes talking is useless; sometimes words are useless.

Chapter XV

Giulia

The phone rings just in the middle of a session with a patient. It is Dr Santini speaking. From her excited and slightly shrill voice I gather that the case is awkward. She isn't excitable in general but, on the contrary, a polite and gentle person. I try to understand what is going on, while waving my hand at the patient sitting in front of me in an apologetic gesture. A girl in the hospital needs an urgent gastroscopy but she refuses to give her consent. They think I can convince her.

My persuasion techniques are required. When they ask for a consultation and time is important I feel the pressure of the patients' anxiety and insecurity, like a gladiator in the arena. Two deep breaths and I take back control of the situation and go on with my patient trying to remember the situation we were analysing. In a few seconds, unconsciously, I start torturing a finger of my right hand and I know what it means.

The session is over, at least for me. I fix a new appointment and then I head to ER.

I see Dr Santini and I ask her about the patient. Dr Santini takes me to a dim room which is, most importantly, far from the voices in ER; it's a perfect room to talk.

She is pale and motionless on the couch; she seems like a fragile, blown glass object that draws your attention and gaze but are not supposed to touch, fearing it could break. I approach her with a smile and introduce myself and her glare, so contrasted with her appearance, hits me.

Dr Santini makes the introductions and says she'll wait elsewhere. I ask the girl what her first name is. In a whisper she says, "Viola." "Unusual name,"

I respond. Her expression tells me she didn't expect this remark and this reaction is significant to me. She does not seem used to compliments, on the contrary, she becomes ironic when somebody praises her. She is not assertive so I go on, following in the wake of my curiosity.

I ask her about her job, family and siblings; friends, hobbies and wishes and dreams; only then do I ask some questions related to her health over the last few days. At first she only answers in monosyllables, then all at once she bursts out: "Why all these questions? When can I go home? What's the use of a gastroscopy?" I look into her eyes and the fighting begins.

"I'd be very glad to say that you could go home but can you assure me that, right now, you could get up, get dressed and take a bus, feeling squashed like a sardine and standing for about half an hour, still finally getting home?"

Viola looks at me with even wider eyes, like a chased animal paralysed by a flash of light at night. Seconds follow that seem endless; I keep looking at her and tears start rolling down her cheeks; now I know we are in tune.

I caress her shoulder to reassure her that such a reaction is alright, the tears, the fear of the test and the emotional turmoil; the high intensity of sensations and the helplessness to understand what's happening are all normal reactions. I try to help her make sense of this tangle of emotions. Viola is a determined person and her confidence is where I start to talk to her from.

The syllogism for her is: Viola does not feel well and not feeling well leads to medical tests, therefore, Viola has to undergo some tests in order to feel well again. I still insist that understanding what makes her feel miserable will help her go back to her life with a positive attitude and with a confidence she doesn't feel now. For the first time Viola covers her face with her hands as if to put away all remaining worries.

I can understand her fears, the test is invasive but not painful. I reassure her by saying that she will be sedated.

Now she should be thinking about the things to come, when everything will be over, and not about the gastroscopy. I suggest to her that she do some relaxation exercises with me. Viola is uncertain and I have to keep reassuring her. Then, reaching a certain point, she looks me straight in the face and says, "I want to take this as a trial of courage."

Chapter XVI

Annamaria

Not that she is fully convinced. The theatre is ready and the girl sedated. I begin with my feet parallel and slightly apart and the endoscope on my shoulder. I insert it; a quick look at the stomach then I get to the duodenum; I take the four bits I need and I align them carefully on the tray to send to the pathologist. I relax. The duodenum shows a possible case of celiac disease. The plicae are pale and undefined. If I get close and squirt some water I can see her intestinal villi or, better still, her horrible villi. Well, she has celiac disease and not a bleeding ulcer. I feel at ease with celiac disease. It is a world I know well. She will be flabbergasted. She will start her gluten-free diet resentfully. She will hate me for a few weeks and then she will feel better. The novelty will fascinate her and she will feel stronger. Then, when feeling better, she will forget how miserable she once felt and again she will want a pizza or a roll with friends. And she will hate me again.

To me it's a normal procedure that I have already been through. It is not the same for her; she'll think she is the only unlucky one in the world.

Moreover, she will have to forget fast food, dinners at friends' (to avoid the embarrassment of explaining the disease) and cakes from the cake shop. She'll be frightened. She will be afraid it is cancer or that she will feel miserable the very moment she eats a piece of 'normal' bread.

Well, yes that is what they say: 'normal bread' and 'normal pasta', meaning that celiac sufferers are not normal and do not eat normal food. And here comes the fictionalised, though still fascinating, story about the early men who were only able to pick fruit and roots, only learning to hunt much later. When they started to grow wheat in the Nile valley not all of them were genetically able to digest it. Of course, those who were, that is: most of the people, saw their health improve. Still a few original ancestors, the great hunters among us, are unable to digest wheat. Thus, the ones now fit to digest wheat are the abnormal ones, because they underwent genetic mutation.

This tale works for a while, especially with young people. Later on they think, despite this story, that they have been unlucky in terms of genetics. Then the next step: so many people would prefer celiac disease to any other. You stay on a diet and that's that. You are all right and are even healthier than the so-called 'normal people.'

Anyway, I am intrigued by celiac disease. It is a fact that the number of people with celiac disease has increased in the last fifty years.

Why? It cannot be a matter of genes since they take thousands of years to mutate. Certainly, the amount of 'gluten' in our diets has increased. Wheat has, if anything, become richer and richer in gluten; the magic protein that makes the dough elastic with bubbles when it leavens.

Besides, it is nourishing. When, as a child, I was very thin, they gave me a kind of small gluten-enriched pasta. A field with this new richer in gluten wheat is worth more both economically and in terms of nutrition. However, the genetic predisposition and gluten aside, there is something else that sets apart the process of celiac disease. We do not know what it is; it might be a virus or a bacterium or different viruses and bacteria that interfere with our immune system turning us into the early men, hunters and berry pickers. I wish I could be that researcher who finds this X factor; I look at the data of my thousand celiac patients over and over. Nothing. I don't have the proper tools to find what causes celiac disease. For a researcher celiac disease proves to be a very good model of study. You eat gluten and get sick. You don't eat it and are almost all right. You eat it again and feel sick again. I don't think other diseases depend on such an on/off switch. Therefore, if we understood what happens in celiac disease, we could also start to understand other diseases we know little about; for instance, joint diseases or chronic bowel inflammations.

My working day is over.

Chapter XVII

Mamma

It's impossible. It is my daughter who tells me why for some months I have felt this sort of tiredness and complacency towards life. Viola is a part of me, just like a tattoo, reminding me that I'm her mother and she is my daughter. Such a bond implies a measure of subordination so that I would have never have fancied her bold enough to tell me about her disease (she is sick, celiac disease, even though she insists in calling it 'food intolerance') and, moreover, to get me off the sofa and to the hospital in order to let a certain doctor do medical tests on me too.

I'm sure she has let herself be persuaded by some odd food theory and yet, she never takes sides.

Since she has known she has celiac disease she has become brave.

In the last few months I've been feeling old, meaning that I no longer care about dinner, that I don't wash regularly, forget the roast in the oven and surrender to Viola as my strength, even the physical one I had just a few years ago, gives way to melancholy, to something I can't pin down but still feel as liberating. I am tired, even tired of talking, and especially to Viola who still makes the wrong choices.

She arrived at an early hour bringing the smell of the street (smog and chips) with her. I left the sofa like a condemned person; I still want to please her but I know she is wrong; I'm going to undergo the tests just to prove to her that, even this time, I'll be right.

I only feel exhaustion and some cramps at night, all normal things at my age.

Indeed, I do not have a good complexion but some makeup will take care of that. Viola is convinced that my symptoms are due to that odd gluten intolerance theory. She is almost pleased to think we share the same genetics as we are totally different in the other things. I'm thoughtful, she is impetuous; I'm committed to cooking, she to books (that gather dust); I'm tall, she isn't; I'm a catholic and she is an atheist.

She takes her father's car. While driving, she rings who knows who, eats a bar (gluten-free of course) and plays the stereo.

It's hot when we get to the hospital. Viola sets the pace, greets people and seems to know everyone on the staff.

She introduces doctors and a tall female doctor in particular: Dr Mancini. She is nice and has a scent of Positano soap; she tells me about the tests and the purpose of them. She says there could be a genetic link between Viola and me, which means that I too, could have celiac disease and so I will make them both happy if I have the tests. In their opinion, the symptoms I've been showing for a number of months are an alarm bell, especially the trembling legs and the inexplicable drowsiness.

Viola comforts me but she'd be better off looking after my bag and clothes; she'd be more useful that way. Viola thinks that fears too are hereditary; crazy, they are not. Fears are only untruthful.

They did all kinds of tests and I'll have a gastroscopy in the afternoon. Viola wanted to wait outside, perhaps as a mark of respect towards my pain, however, she didn't know that a gastroscopy is nothing compared to other pains. A whole day spent with my daughter thanks to the celiac disease. We talked while waiting. She tells me about a new guy and I gather there's a Mr So-and-so she likes because of his bright eyes; she would like to go to Paris because there's an exhibition on of a contemporary artist who paints baby food jars.

"Why," I ask, "do you like such weird things?"

Baby food represents babies; their first meal and their introduction to life. The artist, she explains, collects the jars, which are the first account of life of the adults-to-be and paints landscapes, abstract pictures and rainbows in order to give an image of the child's future life as a present to the baby.

I'm touched and think of Viola's first hunger. She loved eating and used to eat everything. Later, while growing up, she started to eat less and badly, then she almost stopped eating. Now she eats gluten-free food, however, she does eat.

Then we talk about her house. It is terrible. She begins to raise her voice and jumps on me saying that I don't understand anything, then, in a rage, stops talking. When mothers do not understand children should act as interpreters using psychic powers to read minds. If I don't understand, help me, don't stay silent.

Do I have celiac disease? At my age?

Dr Mancini explains that even if you don't have the disease at birth it may develop in time as it is caused by large amounts of gluten taken in over the years. I thought I was depressed but, instead, I have celiac disease.

Viola and I are alike.

Viola interrupts Mancini every two minutes with her talking, she lists the things I can eat, the tests to repeat and the causes of the disease.

I feel confused; it's not easy to change habits at my age. However, as usual, I make her think it will be as easy as walking.

Chapter XVIII

Viola

I can think of nothing else except the disease and what to eat; it has become a sort of obsession.

At first I thought it was nonsense, an absurd idea of Dr Mancini's mind. How could harmless, satisfying and healthy bread (the first food I had loved besides mum's milk) be slowly and implacably killing me? I hadn't realised it, apart my bowel cramps and the runs to the bathroom. The doctor says we cannot know when I developed the disease. If, as she says, the feeling of uneasiness is one of the signs, well, I remember it all along. I remember a trip to the mountains when I was at school and how happy I was. Then I remember the heat on the bus, the sense of nausea always there, even when I sat on a stone, behind the group. That left me with a sensation of being in hell, tired and depressed. "It must be a virus," my mother had said. Since then I have remembered the sensation of being tired, unable to do simple things. Well, I didn't always feel that way; I mean, not every day, but now that I feel well I know it wasn't normal.

When I thought I was 'normal' I lived miserably and now, not being 'normal,' I live happily.

I'd never known what being well, feeling strong and waking up in the morning nice and fresh meant. Now, since I have been on a diet, my thoughts seem to run faster, in confusion and the several sensations mingle like different flavours in a Thai dish do. I wonder why I'm thinking about Thai cooking, probably because of the rice. Anyway, I feel slightly scared by my thoughts because I can't catalogue them as I do with my art books. I still see Dr Castaldi. She says I'm doing well and adapting, that I need time and that celiac disease therapy is very simple; all you need to do is eat gluten-free food.

No grain, no pain. A scientific review with this title was on Santini's desk. I don't think it's true; the authors do not have the disease; there is always some 'pain'. The pain that comes of not savouring the smell and taste of that first bite into crispy toast or a steaming pizza, and the sorrow at the 'never' the doctors keep repeating.

Never again eat pasta, never a sandwich. That's not fair. I have a routine to follow now. I have to go to my doctor's to get the prescription for my pasta, look for well-stocked shops, read the labels of the goods I buy at the supermarket, make my own bread and cakes daily. The sunny side of it is Dr Degiacomo, the chemist. I do like him. He helped me to have a clue among the choice of gluten-free cookies and pastas. I would not describe him as handsome, yet he is young, caring and calm; as good as his plum cakes, as light as bio-yoghurt. I don't feel like going out yet and that says it all. I keep safe in my goldfish bowl like the goldfish I had as a child and look at the world through the opaque glass. I did not go to my colleague's birthday. It was in a restaurant and I wouldn't have known what to order or how to explain it to the others; yes, because, besides living it, we have to tell people about the disease.

However, I meet my mother more often and I am worried about her.

Eating with her is a way to share a meal, the house and a few words. The moment Dr Mancini said 'like mother like daughter' she suddenly turned pale. It was not the news that she had celiac disease that turned her pale but the awareness that her genes had transmitted the disease, the same genes she was so proud of because they had given me the fine features that make us alike.

And she appeared older. She didn't answer, looked numb and I took her home as if in a trance to the safety of her home. Now I look at her through different eyes and our roles are reversed. I am the one who supports her now and read the labels to her.

I am brilliant at making self-made bread: I mix the flour, add herbs, olives, some sugar at times and every day I try a new recipe for mum and me. I want me to like it, I want mum to like it. I can do no more but I'd like to take her to the seaside. A balcony overlooking the sea, a small bar on the beach. Time to ourselves, to test our complete fusion as adults.

Dr Castaldi repeats it at every session, "You need to get into action." This is reality I live in and I won't change it by getting angry or by merely protesting against it. I have to get into action: make my bread, weigh myself and undergo the tests; go buy gluten-free pasta and snacks and cook, inviting my mother to dinner whenever I can. I feel stronger every day, I think that my hair is thicker and that my nails, which are now painted red, have grown stronger.

I'm still slim but I put on 3 kilos and that's not a fancy. My complexion seems clear but not pale.

Most of all I sleep better. I dream of endless wanderings on which I can regain something forgotten or stolen; I am a gold digger, a pilgrim, a globetrotter, a clochard, a beggar. No one comes along with me on the way but I keep walking and searching, then the alarm at 06:30 am and I'm back to reality between the basin and the shower cubicle.

A text arrives, an invitation to an aperitif; it's from Degiacomo who writes, 'Marco.'

I send an, 'ok.'

Write, 'Viola.'

Chapter XIX

Annamaria

"Hello?"

"Hello, is it you Annamaria? Where are you?"

"Giulia! I'm at the airport going to London for a medical convention. Sorry for not telling you, but you know, time is always short. I'll be back at the weekend and, please, send me an e-mail if there's something new." The line moves as I give my greetings.

At the airport I already feel a sense of freedom as my trip begins right there. I immediately feel the coming-and-going atmosphere; there are Americans, Chinese, Poles, Africans and tanned, recently arrived Italians, and Italians with bags under their eyes, ready to board. I did everything I had to: I called my daughter, informed the hospital and left my numbers for urgent messages; bought some magazines I won't finish reading, remembered the battery charger and the mobile battery; brought the PC, the USB stick and the MP3-player (so that I can reflect on Vivaldi's music).

I look for a toilet, not because I need it, but because I like to look at myself in the mirror, to greet myself before boarding. My adult expression surprises me, I can't accept the silver hairs, the wrinkles across my forehead or the eyes, tired from the many hours spent in front of the PC screen.

I stand there and look at myself but what the reflection in the mirror does not show exactly is how I feel.

The mirror doesn't show my fears, my uncertainty and the anger that comes at me when things go wrong, when my mother forgets my birthday, when the elevator to the fifth floor is out of order or when they don't let me express my ideas. So they often stay hidden in the secret places of my life and I forget about them as time passes. The call for my flight comes, I have to go to the gate; I gather my bags and ideas and leave this confessional before someone comes in and finds me with my nose glued to the washbowl mirror.

I'd like everything to be a different way. I'd stay at home, in an armchair and even wearing a training suit and slippers to welcome English, Spanish and Russian; American and Brazilian colleagues. We would sip tea and have cookies while vividly discussing the latest scientific discoveries. I would present my report written on the drawing pad that my little nephew doodles in; celiac disease illustrated with a child's coloured-crayons. I would order pizzas for everybody, for us who are not celiac and go on eating quantities of gluten per month, forgetful of the disease. After all, we are intolerant of other things, of losing time, of standing in line at the cinema, of moaning people.

During my working years I have met many patients, some of whom I remember the voice of or a particular movement of the face; of others it's the look, the posture or the smell of their skin. These people did not feel sick; to my astonishment they lived a normal life though, admittedly, with some limitations such as repeatedly taking tests or depending on drugs. The sick people I have met and the healthy are alike. Sick people, exactly like the healthy ones, watch soap operas, tell jokes and go on holidays with their families; they have political ideas, support voting and get undressed and make love; they enjoy themselves and weep on their children's birthday and are not afraid of losing their life simply because they are living it. Where is the line between sick and healthy people?

We are sick when we don't take care of ourselves and don't enjoy our days; we are sick when we pursue unreachable objectives and forget about the daily victories; when we forget about ourselves, as if our priorities lay elsewhere, other than in our souls. We forget we should give ourselves a small, a very small, but meaningful present every day.

I wander in the airport as in a bazaar. I'm aware I'm playing for time. I head for the exit.

I decide that my trip begins outside the airport; I carry my bag and my feet to a taxi and browbeat the driver into taking me to the national library.

It's early in the morning and there aren't many people in here and this is good for me; the suit I'm wearing and my briefcase don't suit the atmosphere of the place. I ask for the children's' section, I'm looking for a specific book but can hardly remember the author's name. They think I'm nuts. They balk at my request, but then they help, showing me a series of brightly coloured small books and so, by the cover, I recognise the author's style. Here it is! This is his book.

My young patient finished it. I read the book and look at his beautiful drawings, which could only have been done by a knowing and serene hand.

Reading is travel.

A personal, inner kind of travel; that the day belongs only to me and that I'm looking forward to telling someone about it.

Chapter XX

Mamma

    I haven't written to you since you got your high school diploma and that time later when you graduated, I'm afraid of making spelling mistakes; you know, a mother doesn't like her daughter to correct her, especially a mother who has spent millions of minutes correcting and observing every single thing, until almost deafening you.
    I am writing to thank you. Since I've known that I have celiac disease I have known you. I've spent about thirty years with you and, in spite of my motherly attention, I missed some particulars that, as you say, are like the shading in the paintings in your catalogues.
    I'm proud of you. I approve of your job and I don't think it is boring or sad, I envy your accuracy and the head you have always had for remembering dates, codes, authors and facts. Your ability to recognise a painting and its creator from small details moves me. You don't know that when I go and do the shopping and have a chat with the other elderly housewives I revel in extolling your competence; my daughter works in the field of art, my daughter knows all about paintings, their frames and even the walls they have been hung on.
    Now we eat in a better, a healthier way according to celiac disease. I have to say that it has been hard; it hasn't been simple to change my eating habits at my age. On the other hand, having you at home every day and cooking together, has pushed me towards new things and has made choosing and preparing meals easier. I invented a dish and named it 'Viola salad.' Now we have a dish to eat together and we share not only the disease but our chats as well, while eating rice and chicken; they are an elixir of youth because they make me your partner.

We are very similar and not only because of the disease. You never surrender, you love reading and travelling; you are argumentative to the bitter end and you often persevere.

Let it go. Concentrate on what you really care about; you will not feel tired if it is something worthwhile and you will always see results, sometimes unexpected ones.

Love too is unexpected. Don't be afraid of loving.

Do you know why I named you Viola? Once I read that in pre-Roman times, this colour *viola*, purple in English, was linked to famines and thus it came before the 'ver sacrum'; that's why, to Christians, this colour signifies change or renewal.

You were my source of renewal; your birth would mean new life not only because you were starting yours but because becoming a mother was the most important change in my life.

You have been 'viola' again during these months, with the discovery of the disease. My lifestyle, my diet, has changed and been renewed, and I couldn't have done it without you.

Don't see yourself as the ugly duckling. You are lovely; on the balcony when I look at you coming to the door, I see a special light emanating from you. We are lovely unless we are spent and you are worth billions of stars.

I belong to another generation: crying is shameful, cuddles and coaxing useless; and to say 'I love you,' needless between a mother and a child. These days I've been thinking of my love for you and the more I think of it the more I am unable to quantify it.

Now, imagine all the sand on the planet, all the beaches on all the coasts in all the world, count all the grains and think to yourself that my love for you equals them.

May every day be a 'viola' for you, a rebirth, because change means progress and improvement.

We have changed; we got the disease and we improved.

With the love I still have to give and give to you.

Your mum.

Chapter XXI

Viola

A year has passed since the diagnosis. Dr Castaldi was right. You need time, time to adapt; besides, let's put it this way, you need to work on your inside and on your outside.

On the inside because you need overcome the unbalance you have lived with for years, the sense of instability and precariousness that has influenced many of your choices. You have to accept that your being so frail may be due to an undiagnosed illness, to a poison that, every day, was eating your strength up. Work on the outside means to register with the supporting association, to learn how to cook and to read food labels; to organise your shopping so that you don't forget anything and to travel being aware of the restaurants and shops available to you. Luckily, we have the web and luckily The Celiac Association is there to help me when I'm down. They always have something to propose. Always a gentle word for anyone who calls. Today it is my birthday. It's a Saturday and I have arranged a picnic at Villa Borghese.

The menu is gluten-free but my guests don't know. A challenge to pizzas and sandwiches. Salty crepes, vegetable filled bundles and fruit sticks even a cake with cream and strawberries made with cornmeal and rice flour by my mother. A grand gourmet menu that my mother and I prepared. I get dressed. I'm happy; I can see my future and I like it. They will all be there, Dr Degiacomo and, even better, Marco too, which is why I am putting on my mascara.

Chapter XXII

Readers' Guide

This novel was written to focus on patients' perspectives on some relevant aspects of celiac disease and to give caregivers' perspectives on related issues.

The novel is about celiac disease for two reasons. Firstly, celiac disease is an emerging disease, so frequent as to be considered a 'social epidemic' and it involves several interventions, besides the medical one. Secondly, we, the writers, know celiac disease well because we have been working for many years with celiac patients (CC and MS) and/or because we have already been involved with professional writing on celiac disease and food-related disorders (TB).

The story is about a common case, not a real one but a representative one.

A young woman, whose symptoms become worse and worse until, eventually, a diagnosis is made.

Celiac disease is not rare and we have to face this fact in order to make a correct diagnosis. Not only doctors should consider it but also patients, who, can help make the diagnosis themselves. Indeed, there are cases in which the patient himself 'suggests' to the doctor the possibility of him having a food intolerance and, in particular, celiac disease.

A diagnosis of celiac disease is a great opportunity to improve a person's life because the prescribed diet improves their health and, in turn, the overall quality of their life.

However, it isn't always that we agree with the saying *'no grain, no pain.'* Adaptation to a limited diet can be difficult. Several studies have indicated that the key to a successful adaptation to celiac disease is through obtaining a thorough knowledge of it and being aware that support groups can be of a great help. A personal inclination towards tolerance and compliance, as far as the new situation goes, has also been found to be essential. An excessively easy-going attitude that might result in frequent dietary lapses can, however, be dangerous for the health. Therefore, it is very helpful to maintain a constant relationship with the healthcare advisers at a dedicated clinic; they can help you to adapt and to maintain the correct attitude to living with celiac disease.

The aim of this novel is to offer a simple tool that can be used to increase knowledge of celiac disease and to 'humanise', as much as possible, what is often seen as an extraordinary event.

We are confident that the increasing knowledge of many of the aspects of celiac disease will eventually fill the gap between the expected prevalence of the disease (that is the number of persons that will develop celiac disease, even if they do not recognise it) and the number of those who receive an actual diagnosis of the disease. And last but not least, we believe that a diagnosis of celiac disease can grant an opportunity to change for better and grant a greater life expectancy. Unfortunately, one cannot expect this from most chronic diseases; that's why celiac disease differs from other chronic illnesses. A celiac sufferer without the time or will to become aware of celiac disease and the gluten-free world, who is unable to reach the health care and advocacy group they need, will mostly experience celiac disease as a burden and will not benefit from the changes that could have been made for a better life. It is the responsibility of those who care for CD patients to use all the available tools to disseminate the knowledge of the disease itself and of the tricks to ease the burden by, for example, choosing the right food, avoiding gluten and sometimes renouncing one's favourite food. Therefore, this novel is our small contribution to the vast and ever expanding celiac world.

Chapter XXIII

Medical Notes

Note 1

Viola is a young woman who has been experiencing abdominal symptoms for months. She reports an increase in the frequency of bowel movements and an urgent need of evacuation soon after a meal. She also feels the bothersome sensations of bloating and distension in her abdomen. She has lost some weight, which may have been caused by a reduction of food intake due to fear of increasing the diarrhoea. She always feels tired and irritable. She is of the impression that she has a poor quality of life.

What do Viola's symptoms suggest?

Gastrointestinal symptoms are quite common in young adults and are often related to a disorder called irritable bowel syndrome. This was the diagnosis that Viola had when the story began. Irritable bowel syndrome patients do not show up as any different to celiac disease sufferers in the usual laboratory tests and even more sophisticated examinations, such as an endoscopy, may not show it. In the Western World the rate is high in the general population and the number of women almost doubles the number of men.

The diagnosis is made according to the so called Rome III criteria: recurrent abdominal pain or discomfort at least 3 days/month in the last 3 months associated with two or more of the following: improvement with defecation, onset associated with a change in frequency of stool, onset associated with a change in form (appearance) of stool. Irritable bowel syndrome is considered a 'functional disease' because no apparent alteration is found in the bowel.

The familiar occurrence of irritable bowel syndrome suggests the possibility of a genetic predisposition but also some food containing sugars that you can't absorb (milk, vegetables and fruit) as well as psychological factors may play a role. However, patients suffering from an irritable bowel may have an undiagnosed food intolerance. It is now recommended that patients with irritable bowel syndrome also be tested for milk intolerance and celiac disease. These two intolerances are the most common food intolerances in the Western World.

References

Drossman, D.A., Corazziari, E., Delvaux, M., Talley, N.J., Thompson, W.G., Spiller, R.C., Whitehead, W.E., eds. *The functional gastrointestinal disorders: diagnosis, pathophysiology and treatment. A multinational consensus.* 3rd ed. McLean, V.A.: Degnon Associates, 2006.

Sperber, A.D., Drossman, D.A., and Quigley, E.M. The global perspective on irritable bowel syndrome: a Rome Foundation-World Gastroenterology Organisation symposium. *Am J Gastroenterol*, 2012. 107(11): p. 1602.

Note 2

Viola is admitted to emergency because she fainted; eventually, she was found to have anaemia due to an iron deficiency. In her medical history Viola reports fatigue and gastrointestinal symptoms.

Why was Viola suspected to have celiac disease?

Anaemic patients may experience fainting, which is, in medical terminology, a: *vasovagal syncope*.

This event is most frequently due to acute blood loss and this is the reason for which Viola was promptly admitted to the hospital and needed to undergo an endoscopy. It is rarely due to chronic anaemia. In the case of Viola the high temperature in the shop, the crowd and brisk movement may have stimulated the vagus nerve, excess acetylcholine was released, the heart rate slowed and the blood vessels dilated, making it harder for blood to defeat gravity and be pumped to the brain. This temporary decrease in blood flow to the brain causes the syncopal (fainting) episode.

When the clinical records were revised it became apparent that longstanding gastrointestinal symptoms, severe iron deficiency and consequent anaemia required a search for the cause of the blood loss or, as an alternative, chronic iron malabsorption. An upper endoscopy was mandatory to ascertain the presence of gastrointestinal bleeding (from a gastric or duodenal ulcers, or an erosive gastritis, that can occur after anti-inflammatory drugs use). The upper endoscopy consists of the insertion, by the mouth, under sedation, of a tube that allows the view of the inner lining of the oesophagus, stomach and duodenum. It also allows for the taking of biopsies, samples of mucosa that can be analysed by a pathologist. In the case of Viola, no bleeding sites were detected and the appearance of the duodenal mucosa was suggestive of celiac disease. In fact, the normal appearance of the duodenal mucosa is that of a bright pink velveteen liner that, in the case of inflammation, such as active celiac disease, loses its brightness and appears 'scalloped.'

Iron is absorbed in the first tract of the duodenum. An inflammation of the duodenal mucosa may put at risk the absorption of iron and cause a progressive decrease of iron stores and levels of haemoglobin even without any bleeding.

References

Card, T.R., et al., An excess of prior irritable bowel syndrome diagnoses or treatments in Celiac disease: evidence of diagnostic delay. *Scand J Gastroenterol*, 2013. Jul; 48(7): 801-7.

Note 3

Viola is eventually diagnosed with celiac disease.

What is celiac disease?

Celiac disease is food intolerance. In particular, celiac disease is an intolerance of wheat, barley, rye and whey. In most of the world cereals and above all wheat, are the main source of carbohydrates in a person's diet some examples of which are: bread, pasta, pizza and cookies. Wheat and the other cereals, mentioned above, contain proteins that are commonly called *gluten*, that have been proven to retain, upon digestion, fragments that are toxic to some individuals. In fact, in genetically predisposed individuals, (a figure of about 1 person out of 100) the ingestion of gluten causes an immune-mediated reaction that leads to a variable degree of inflammation of the inner lining of the intestine and a rise in the blood of a number of antibodies. Antibodies are proteins generated during the immune response that, through the blood stream, reach and damage organs and tissues far from the intestine. For this reason celiac disease is considered an autoimmune disorder, that implies that the body of the person with celiac disease who eats gluten, in the attempt to mount a defence against it, produce antibodies that not only attack gluten but also his/her body.

Celiac disease may go undiscovered for years, and patients have often been judged by family members and doctors as being effected by imaginary symptoms while they feel fatigued, have recurrent abdominal distress and generally perceive themselves to have a low quality of life.

The onset of symptoms that characterise celiac disease vary from case to case. There is the possibility that gastrointestinal symptoms or a failure to thrive appear in a child after weaning, i.e. a few weeks or months after the first ingestion of gluten. But celiac disease may also appear in young adults and in older persons, more frequently (almost double the number) in women. In adults, gastrointestinal symptoms are present in less than 50% of cases. Other common symptoms are fatigue, depression and irritability; infertility can also be a symptom. It is common to find the following in lab test results: an iron deficiency, low lipids, and proteins, as well as abnormal liver function. The reason for the wide variability of the onset and clinical presentation of the disease is, at the moment, not fully understood. The current hypothesis is that other triggers besides genetics and the ingestion of gluten, such as an infection, for example, may play a role.

For unclear reasons the prevalence of celiac disease has risen significantly in the past decades. One US study found that over 50 years there has been a fourfold increase in the prevalence of celiac disease, with another study from Finland reporting a twofold increase (Rubio-Tapia 2009; Lohi 2007).

References

Ludvigsson, J.F., Leffler, D.A., Bai, J.C., Biagi, F., Fasano, A., Green, P.H., Hadjivassiliou, M., Kaukinen, K., Kelly, C.P., Leonard, J.N., Lundin, K.E., Murray, J.A., Sanders, D.S., Walker, M.M., Zingone, F., Ciacci, C. The Oslo definitions for celiac disease and related terms. *Gut*, 2013. 62(1): p. 43-52.

Murch, S., Jenkins, H., Auth, M., Bremner, R., Butt, A., France, S., Furman, M., Gillett, P., Kiparissi, F., Lawson, M., McLain, B., Morris, M.A., Sleet, S., Thorpe, M. Joint BSPGHAN and Celiac UK guidelines for the diagnosis and management of celiac disease in children. *Arch Dis Child*. 2013 Oct; 98(10): 806-11.

Rubio-Tapia, A., Hill, I.D., Kelly, C.P., Calderwood, A.H., Murray, J.A.; American College of Gastroenterology. ACG clinical guidelines: diagnosis and management of celiac disease. *Am J Gastroenterol*. 2013 May; 108(5): 656-76.

Note 4

How common is celiac disease and what symptoms warn of the presence of it?

Screening studies performed in many countries indicate that celiac disease is found in the general population in about 1 person out of every 100. However, some diseases and symptoms are frequently associated with celiac disease. Therefore, in certain cases, the frequency of celiac disease may be higher than 1:100. For example, testing for celiac disease is highly recommended in patients with gastrointestinal symptoms and/or in cases of iron deficiency. Out of those people who suffer with gastrointestinal symptoms the prevalence may rise to 1 out of 10. Once it is suspected, a diagnosis of celiac disease is made by searching for specific antibodies in the blood. It is best if the blood test is performed before any food restriction is started, namely: while not on a gluten-free diet. The blood tests include the search for the antibodies *anti-tissue transglutaminase IgA* (a-TTG) and *immunoglobulin IgA* and are eventually followed by the *antiendomysium antibody* test. All are highly appropriate, being specific indicators of the presence of celiac disease. The second step is to confirm the diagnosis with an *intestinal biopsy* that is performed during an esophagogastroduodenoscopy.

A person's test results, which otherwise show the symptoms of celiac disease, might, in unusual circumstances, not show the presence of the above mentioned antibodies in their blood.. In such cases the doctor will prescribe an upper endoscopy with a biopsy of the duodenal mucosa. In fact, damage to the intestinal mucosa suggests a possible gluten intolerance. A second biopsy after a period of gluten-free diet, showing the healing of the intestinal mucosa, will confirm the diagnosis.

References

Reilly, N.R., Fasano, A., Green, P.H. Presentation of celiac disease. *Gastrointest. Endosc Clin N Am.* 2012 Oct; 22(4): 613-2.

Note 5

Viola is experiencing a big change in her life. The first step towards health for her is to adopt a strict gluten-free diet.

What is a gluten-free diet?

The main, fundamental, treatment for celiac disease is the withdrawal of gluten from the diet.

The gluten avoidance has to be total; complete avoidance of gluten, in the case of celiac disease, is always the best. This means for most people with celiac disease adaptation to a new diet in which bread, pasta and pizzas as well as muffins and cakes are forbidden.

Gluten-free food can be divided into food that is naturally gluten-free (rice, corn, potatoes, quinoa, etc.) and commercially available food that has been designed to substitute foods to be avoided but is free from gluten (gluten-free pasta, bread, cakes, cookies, etc.). In most countries, commercially available food can be labelled as gluten-free if the gluten content is no more than 20 parts per million.

Adapting to the new diet can sometimes be challenging because celiac sufferers must think about the composition of every meal and every bite they take apart from their regular meals. They need to plan the purchase of safe gluten-free food in a way that safe food is always available at home, in their offices and on their person if they are travelling. In restaurants and fast food outlets they have to ensure that gluten-free meals are available or that they choose naturally gluten-free food (plain rice, meat, fish, vegetables and fruit) making sure that it is not, for example, cooked in a sauce or in bread crumbs that might contain wheat or other unsafe cereals.

Some celiac sufferers report a restriction on their social lives because of the fear of gluten contamination. In most cases a careful choice of food allows celiac sufferers to eat safely with friends and in restaurants and to continue to have a normal social life.

At the beginning the change is not simple. Women, when compared to men, apparently feel the burden of celiac disease more. They are more often in charge of the shopping, the cooking and the taking care of the children. However, as for many life changes, a certain amount of commitment helps. For example, a good knowledge of food composition, a slight improvement in cooking skills and practice at reading food labels during grocery shopping will all facilitate the task.

A great help comes from patient support groups which are active in all countries. They may indicate places where gluten-free food is available all over the world, provide useful tips for everyday life and offer the support of shared experience.

Note 6

After Viola's diagnosis of celiac disease her mother is also found to have the disease.

Is celiac disease a genetic disease?

Celiac disease often runs in the family. There is a genetic susceptibility that distinguishes people who may be diagnosed with celiac disease at some point in their lives (about 30% of the general population in the Western World) from those who will never have the disease. At the moment we know most, though not all, of the genetics connected with celiac disease.

Our cells bear a class of protein called HLA that recognises fragments of proteins and can trigger the immune response that leads to the production of inflammatory cells, the production of chemical agents (that increase the inflammation) and of antibodies.

Celiac disease patients bear the genes that produce the HLA DQ2 and HLA DQ8 molecules that recognise and bind fragments of ingested gluten causing the production of lymphocytes. Lymphocytes are cells that are responsible for the inflammation and that initiate the chain of events that results in damage to the mucosa, to the intestine and to the production of antibodies. The antibodies, produced during this inflammation, include TTG and EMA and it is their presence in the blood allows for the diagnosis of celiac disease.

Many studies have shown that celiac disease runs in the family. First degree relatives of a celiac sufferer (parents, brothers and sisters) face a risk, that is ten times higher than that of the general population, of developing celiac disease and, in the case of homozygote twins, it is even higher. It is advisable that once a diagnosis is made, all the first degree relatives of a celiac sufferer undergo the blood test to screen for celiac disease.

Note 7

Viola, once diagnosed with celiac disease, experiences a deep change and notices a general improvement in her quality of life.

Is it common for a celiac sufferer to experience such an improvement when adopting the gluten-free diet?

In general, withdrawing gluten and maintaining a strict gluten-free diet leads to the healing of the intestinal mucosa and a progressive decrease in the blood of TTG and EMA until, eventually, they disappear.

The process may be rapid for some and most symptoms disappear within a few weeks, however, it may be slower for others and can take months or even years. In rare cases symptoms do not improve and the blood test does not normalise. The doctor will first make sure that the diagnosis of celiac disease was correct and then investigate for the causes of the persistence of symptoms. Celiac disease may not exclude the presence of irritable bowel syndrome and, most of the time, gastrointestinal symptoms that do not improve with a strict gluten-free diet may be related to that. However, other causes beside irritable bowel syndrome should also be investigated. The most severe, albeit very rare, complication of celiac disease is enteropathy associated lymphoma.

Celiac disease patients on a gluten-free diet also experience an improvement in the quality of their sleep, a better sexual relationship with their partner(s) and a general improvement to their quality of life.

References

Barratt, S.M., Leeds, J.S., Sanders, D.S. Quality of life in Celiac Disease is determined by perceived degree of difficulty adhering to a gluten-free diet, not the level of dietary adherence ultimately achieved. *J Gastrointestin Liver Dis*. 2011 Sep; 20(3): 241-5.

de Rosa, A., Troncone, A., Vacca, M., Ciacci, C. Characteristics and quality of illness behaviour in celiac disease. *Psychosomatics*. 2004 Jul-Aug; 45(4): 336-42.

Fera, T., Cascio, B., Angelini, G., Martini, S., Guidetti, C.S. Affective disorders and quality of life in adult celiac disease patients on a gluten-free diet. *Eur J Gastroenterol Hepatol*. 2003 Dec; 15(12): 1287-92.

Norström, F., Lindholm, L., Sandström, O., Nordyke, K., Ivarsson, A. Delay to celiac disease diagnosis and its implications for health-related quality of life. *BMC Gastroenterol*. 2011 Nov 7 ;11:118..

Sainsbury, K., Mullan, B., Sharpe, L. Gluten-free diet adherence in celiac disease. The role of psychological symptoms in bridging the intention-behaviour gap. *Appetite*. 2013 Feb; 61(1): 52-8.

Note 8

Viola was admitted to the hospital in what seemed to be a life-threatening condition.

Is celiac disease a life-threatening disease?

No, celiac disease, in the vast majority of cases, is not a life–threatening disease. In rare cases diarrhoea or anaemia, if not promptly corrected, may be of some risk related to dehydration and insufficient oxygenation of tissues.

However, patients with undiagnosed, and to lesser extent diagnosed celiac disease, have been shown to have a higher mortality rate than those with negative serology for celiac disease.

These mortality figures are due to the fact that untreated celiac disease is considered a premalignant condition. Several studies indicate that the inflammation of the intestinal mucosa due to gluten ingestion increases the risk of cancer in the celiac sufferer and in particular the T cell lymphoma.

The increased mortality rates decrease with the years on a gluten-free diet and, 5 years after diagnosis, the risk of death for a celiac sufferer is identical to a non-celiac one, meaning that a gluten-free diet induces recovery of intestinal damage and protects from cancer.

References

Lebwohl, B., Granath, F., Ekbom, A., Smedby, K.E., Murray, J.A., Neugut, A.I., Green, P.H., Ludvigsson, J.F. Mucosal healing and risk for lymphoproliferative malignancy in celiac disease: a population-based cohort study. *Ann Intern Med.* 2013 Aug 6; 159(3): 169-75.

Ludvigsson, J.F., Leslie, L.A., Lebwohl, B., Neugut, A.I., Gregory, M.J., Bhagat, G., Green, P.H. Incidence of lymphoproliferative disorders in patients with celiac disease. *Am J Hematol.* 2012 Aug; 87(8): 754-9.

Rubio-Tapia, A., Kyle, R.A., Kaplan, E.L., Johnson, D.R., Page, W., Erdtmann, F., Brantner, T.L., Kim, W.R., Phelps, T.K., Lahr, B.D., Zinsmeister, A.R., Melton, L.J. 3rd, Murray, J.A. Increased prevalence and mortality in undiagnosed celiac disease. *Gastroenterology.* 2009 Jul; 137(1): 88-93.

West, J., Logan, R.F., Smith, C.J., Hubbard, R.B., Card, T.R. (2004) Malignancy and mortality in people with celiac disease: population based cohort study. *BMJ* 329: 716–719.

Note 9

Viola has conflicting feelings about her life with celiac disease. Before diagnosis she was feeling tired and depressed. She was worried and anxious because of her gastrointestinal symptoms and her tiredness.

What are the possible feelings of an adult person diagnosed with celiac disease?

Before diagnosis Viola was experiencing a mix of feelings in part due to poor health status and in part to a depressive state. In particular, she was suffering from the inability to enjoy the activities she was engaged in and lacked the motivation or desire to engage in any activity ("motivational anhedonia"). She was also suffering from excessive worry, a feeling of not being useful and felt she was unable to deal with everyday life. Therefore, she was feeling a mix of depression and anxiety.

Feelings of depression and anxiety are common in undiagnosed celiac disease patients. Whether this is a symptom of the disease itself or the effect of a disequilibrium due to the lack of health or poor wellbeing without a clear diagnosis of the disease, is still unknown. Feeling depressed influences familial and working relationships but also the quality of sleep, the person who is depressed can, for example, suffer from early awaking and insomnia. Essentially, depression affects one's entire personal life.

However, anxiety is also frequently found to be present before a diagnosis of celiac disease has been made. Anxiety can manifest itself in a variety of ways, including; feelings of fear, worry and some physical symptoms such as palpitations, being short of breath, nausea and nervous tremours. Feelings of anxiety are made up of several components: the cognitive component, which is mainly composed of tense expectance of an undesirable event. The body is ready to face this peril with a reactive behaviour that is characterised by high blood pressure and an increased heart rate; an increase in sweating and dilated pupils. Behaviour may change in the individual's attempts to escape from the perceived conditions of their anxiety. These changes are the main sign of a non-adaptive behaviour although anxiety is not to be considered as a pathological state but a common feeling that is important to human desire in the sense that it helps us to survive and overcome difficult situations.

After a diagnosis of CD has been made and treatment, in the form of the gluten-free diet has started, feelings of anxiety have been shown to progressively reduce in intensity and, eventually, disappear in the vast majority of cases. This is certainly due to the fact that CD is a benign disease and, indeed, is considered by some to 'not even [be] a disease, just a food intolerance' but also because of the progressive disappearance of symptoms and a general improvement in the health of the patient.

Tiredness and fatigue are common in celiac patients. Patients tend to perceive fatigue as a term that encompasses suffering from aching muscles, a lack of strength, irritability and a bodily weakness that interferes with the activity of everyday life.

As a symptom, fatigue is the result of a complex control system of energy output that encompasses hormones, neural transmission, cognitive processing and sensory input. It is frequently reported in primary care and can be related to systemic or neuromuscular disease. In the case of a celiac patient it may also be related to poor sleep patterns that improve with the dietetic treatment.

However, in some circumstances, even the most skilled celiac sufferer will feel the burden of celiac disease. At a party, in a restaurant, on a journey or in a foreign country celiac patients may experience the loneliness of his/her condition, the difficulty of explaining that 'bread is toxic to me.' As circumstances will generate feelings of anger and sadness a consultation with a psychologist may be necessary.

The role of the psychologist/psychiatrist is to help the celiac patient to distinguish between expected functional feelings of sadness and frustration from feelings that will be detrimental to overcoming the change (depression, guilt and anxiety). It is also recommended that expert personnel train the celiac patient how to employ adaptive strategies and problem-solving strategies and not to avoid these forms of useful behaviour.

References

Addolorato, G., Mirijello, A., D'Angelo, C., et al. State and trait anxiety and depression in patients affected by gastrointestinal diseases: psychometric evaluation of 1641 patients referred to an internal medicine outpatient setting. *Int J Clin Pract* 2008; 62: 1063–9.

Arigo, D., Anskis, A.M., Smyth, J.M. Psychiatric comorbidities in women with celiac disease. *Chronic Illn.* 2012 Mar; 8 (1): 45-55.

Ciacci, C., et al., Depressive symptoms in adult celiac disease. *Scand J Gastroenterol*, 1998. 33(3): p. 247-50.
Seligman, Walker & Rosenhan, 2001 *Diagnostic and Statistical Manual of Mental Disorders*, Fourth Edition (DSM-IV).
Siniscalchi, M., Iovino, P., Tortora, R., Forestiero, S., Somma, A., Capuano, L., Franzese, M.D., Sabbatini, F. & Cliacci, C. Fatigue in adult celiac disease. *Aliment Pharmacol Ther* 2005; 22: 489–494.
Smith, D.F., Gerdes, L.U. Meta-analysis on anxiety and depression in adult celiac disease. *Acta Psychiatr Scand.* 2012 Mar;125(3):189-93.
Zingone, F., Siniscalchi, M., Capone, P., Tortora, R., Andreozzi, P., Capone, E., Ciacci, C.. The quality of sleep in patients with celiac disease. *Aliment Pharmacol Ther.* 2010 Oct; 32(8): 1031-6.

Note 10

One of our characters in Chapter 9 tells the doctor that although celiac disease was eliminated in diagnosis he still feels good when avoiding gluten even though he is a cook and being on a gluten-free diet interferes with his work. He does not understand the difference between the general health benefits of a gluten-free diet and yet not having celiac disease. He has been told that he has a non-celiac gluten sensitivity.

What is non-celiac gluten sensitivity?

An increasing number of people diagnosed as not having celiac disease report remission of gastrointestinal and non-gastrointestinal symptoms after removal of gluten from their diet. This condition has been given the name, by contemporaries, of non-celiac gluten sensitivity.

There is some dissonance between the increasing number of patients with non-celiac gluten sensitivity and the fact that, until recently, no unusual biomarker has been found in their blood or intestines.

As matter of fact, the existence of non-celiac gluten sensitivity, is still a subject of debate among scientists. Some data seems to indicate that in non-celiac gluten sensitivity cases there is an abortive response to gluten for which the inflammatory reaction is not fully triggered, therefore the biopsy will not show the presence of intestinal damage. Although anti-endomysium antibodies and antitransglutaminase antibodies are not present, antigliadin antibodies have been found in the blood of about 50% of patients reporting improvement in their symptoms when on a gluten-free diet despite the fact that celiac disease has been excluded.

Recent data shows that, in some cases, the removal of food rich in non-absorbable sugars from the diet may improve their symptoms independent of any effects gluten may or may not have. The non-absorbable sugars are fructose, maltose and polyols which are found in fruit and vegetables; lactose being the sugar present in milk.

A recent study by our group has shown that more than 40% of patients with a non-celiac gluten sensitivity, also commonly do not include in their diet, besides gluten: milk and dairy products, preserved meats, nuts and, in terms of fruit, apples and pears.

It must be noted that the gluten-free diet, although expensive and demanding, is not harmful to non-celiac sufferers if the nutritional content of that diet is well-balanced.

Further studies, and particularly long-term clinical trials in a large number of patients, will make it clear if a gluten-free diet is really necessary for non-celiac gluten sensitivity and if gluten is the main or only trigger of the symptoms. It will also clarify if there is a possibility of reducing the amount of gluten in the diet or of returning, after a while, to a diet that contains gluten.

References

Catassi, C., Bai, J.C., Bonaz, B., Bouma, G., Calabrò, A., Carroccio, A., Castillejo, G., Ciacci, C., Cristofori, F., Dolinsek, J., Francavilla, R., Elli, L., Green, P., Holtmeier, W., Koehler, P., Koletzko, S., Meinhold, C., Sanders, D., Schumann, M., Schuppan, D., Ullrich, R., Vécsei, A., Volta, U., Zevallos, V., Sapone, A., Fasano, A.. Non-celiac gluten sensitivity: the new frontier of gluten related disorders. *Nutrients.* 2013 Sep 26; 5(10): 3839-53.

DiGiacomo, D.V., Tennyson, C.A., Green, P.H., Demmer, R.T. Prevalence of gluten-free diet adherence among individuals without celiac disease in the USA: results from the Continuous National Health and Nutrition Examination Survey 2009-2010. *Scand J Gastroenterol.* 2013 Aug; 48(8): 921-5.

Note 11

The doctor and the psychologist of this novel work in a dedicated clinic for food intolerance and celiac disease.

It is necessary for a celiac sufferer to refer to a dedicated clinic and/or join a patient support group?

Celiac disease is a complex disease in which the management of gastrointestinal and non-gastrointestinal symptoms, of psychological factors and dietetic issues may be better addressed in a dedicated clinic.

A MD that specialises in gastrointestinal disease, an experienced dietitian and a psychologist are all critical to the diagnosis and management of celiac disease. While the necessity for a medical doctor remains for the diagnosis and following procedures for celiac disease, the presence in a clinic of a psychologist has been shown, by the studies, to lead to altered psychological behaviour in celiac patients both before and after diagnosis and dietetic treatment at a very high frequency. Diagnosis of depression and anxiety are common. Moreover, individuals newly diagnosed with celiac disease may experience some uncertainty during the change from their habitual diet to a gluten-free diet and the dietitian support and advice provided will ease this process of adaptation.

References

Baiardini, I., Braido, F., Menoni, S., Bellandi, G., Savi, E., Canonica, G.W., Macchia, D. Wellbeing, illness perception and coping strategies in Italian Celiac patients. *Int J Immunopathol Pharmacol.* 2012 Oct-Dec; 25(4): 1175-82.

Ciacci, C., et al., Psychological dimensions of celiac disease: toward an integrated approach. *Dig Dis Sci,* 2002. 47(9): p. 2082-7.

Ludvigsson, J.F., Green PH. Clinical management of celiac disease. *J Intern Med.* 2011 Jun; 269(6): 560-71.

Smith, M.M., Goodfellow, L. The relationship between quality of life and coping strategies of adults with celiac disease adhering to a gluten-free diet. *Gastroenterol Nurs.* 2011 Nov-Dec; 34(6): 460-8.

Note 12

Annamaria feels tired and stressed and believes she may suffer from burn–out syndrome.

What is burn-out syndrome?

Burn-out syndrome has been defined as a process generating stress typical of care professions (nurses, psychologists, physicians, social workers, priests, etc.).

When inevitable personal stress is added to that of other people's in critical working conditions the result is the burn-out syndrome. The caregiver feels tired and worn out. The resulting irritability interferes with their professional relationships and the person experiencing the burn-out feels deeply dissatisfied.

References

Potter, B. (1994). *Beating Job Burnout. How to transform work pressure into productivity.* Ronin Publishing, Berkeley, California.

Authors' Contact Information

Dr. Tiziana Beato
Writer
tiziana.beato@gmail.com

Dr. Carolina Ciacci
Professor
Chief of Celiac Centre Gastroenterology
University of Salerno
Via S. Allende 43 84081, Italy
cciacci@unisa.it

Dr. Monica Siniscalchi
Adjuct Psychologist
Celiac Center
University of Salerno
Via S. Allende 43 84081, Italy
monicasiniscalchi@alice.it

Index

A

acetylcholine, 55
acid, 8, 15
acne, 9
adaptation, 51, 58, 67
adults, 36, 40, 56, 67
advocacy, 52
age, 35, 36, 37, 47
allergy, 2
ancestors, 34
anger, 43, 64
antibody, 58
anti-inflammatory drugs, 55
anxiety, 4, 25, 29, 31, 63, 64, 65, 67
apples, 66
appointments, 15
assault, 29
atmosphere, 43, 44
avoidance, 58
awareness, 40

B

bacteria, 3, 20, 34
bacterium, 34
benefits, 65
benign, 64
bias, 5
biopsy, 58, 65
blame, 1
bleeding, 24, 29, 33, 55
blood, 5, 9, 20, 23, 25, 54, 57, 58, 60, 65, 66
blood flow, 55
blood stream, 56
blood vessels, 55
bones, 7
bowel, 2, 10, 18, 19, 34, 39, 53, 54, 61
brain, 5, 24, 55
breathing, 22
brittle hair, 29
brothers, 60
burn, 26
burn-out syndrome, 68

C

cancer, 33, 62
carbohydrates, 56
caregivers, 51
cash, 8
Celiac Association, 49
Celiac Disease, 61
cheese, 18
chemical, 60
chicken, 19, 47
children, 2, 19, 36, 44, 57, 59
Christians, 48

chronic diseases, 52
chronic illness, 52
claustrophobic, 25
clinical presentation, 56
clinical trials, 66
coffee, vii, 1, 2, 5, 15, 16
cognitive process, 64
cognitive processing, 64
coke, 19
colon, 20
common symptoms, 56
compliance, 51
composition, 59
consensus, 54
consent, 29, 31
contamination, 59
convention, 43
cooking, 36, 39, 47, 59
coping strategies, 67
cost, 14
cough, 3
crises, 19
criticism, 15
customers, 10, 11, 14

D

defecation, 53
defence, 56
deficiency, 54, 55, 56, 57
dehydration, 62
depression, 56, 63, 64, 65, 67
Diagnostic and Statistical Manual of Mental
    Disorders, 65
diet, 10, 20, 33, 34, 39, 48, 51, 56, 58, 59, 60,
    61, 62, 64, 65, 66, 67
digestion, 56
discomfort, 53
diseases, 5, 34, 57, 64
disequilibrium, 63
disorder, 53, 56
dissonance, 65
distortions, 5
distress, 56
doctors, vii, 15, 21, 23, 26, 27, 36, 40, 51, 56

dough, 34
drawing, 44
dream, 41
drugs, 44
duodenal ulcer, 55
duodenum, 33, 55
dusts, 17

E

elixir of youth, 47
e-mail, 43
embolism, 6
emergency, 21, 54
endoscope, 28, 33
endoscopy, 53, 54, 55, 58
energy, 10, 64
epidemic, 51
equipment, 21
erosive gastritis, 55
esophagogastroduodenoscopy, 58
ethics, 13
evacuation, 2, 53
everyday life, 59, 63, 64
evidence, 55
examinations, 53

F

failure to thrive, 56
fainting, 54, 55
families, 44
family members, 56
fast food, 33, 59
fear(s), 8, 17, 20, 25, 29, 32, 36, 43, 53, 59, 63
feelings, 63, 64
films, 19
Finland, 57
first degree relative, 60
fish, 59
flight, 44
flour, 40, 49
flowers, 2, 25

food, vii, 7, 9, 10, 13, 17, 19, 20, 33, 35, 36, 39, 49, 51, 52, 53, 54, 56, 58, 59, 64, 66, 67
food intake, 53
force, vii
fragments, 56, 60
France, 57
freedom, 9, 21, 43
friendship, 14
fructose, 66
fusion, 40

G

gambling, 1
gastroenterologist, 9
gastrointestinal bleeding, 55
general knowledge, 8
genes, 34, 40, 60
genetic disease, 59
genetic predisposition, 34, 54
genetics, 34, 35, 56, 60
glasses, 5, 7, 9
gravity, 2, 55
guidelines, 57
guilt, 64
guilty, 7, 21, 23

H

hacking, 3
hair, 8, 10, 19, 23, 40
happiness, 10
healing, 3, 58, 60, 62
health, 32, 34, 51, 52, 58, 61, 63, 64, 65
health care, 52
health status, 63
heart rate, 55, 63
helplessness, 32
high blood pressure, 63
HLA, 60
hobby, 13, 14
homozygote, 60
hormones, 64
host, 19

human, 1, 2, 8, 63
husband, 4, 13
hypothesis, 56

I

image, 36
immune response, 56, 60
immune system, 34
immunoglobulin, 58
improvements, 15
individuals, 56, 66, 67
infection, 18, 56
infertility, 56
inflammation, 55, 56, 60, 62
inflammatory cells, 60
ingestion, 56, 62
insane, 9
insecurity, 31
insertion, 55
insomnia, 63
intestinal villi, 33
intestine, 56, 60
iron, 54, 55, 56, 57
irritability, 56, 64, 68
irritable bowel syndrome, 53, 54, 55, 61
issues, 51, 67
Italy, 69

L

laboratory tests, 53
lactose, 66
landscapes, 36
lead, 67
learning, 33
legs, 2, 22, 27, 36
life changes, 59
life expectancy, 52
light, 11, 15, 23, 32, 40, 48
lipids, 56
liver, 56
loneliness, 16, 64
love, 2, 7, 13, 18, 21, 44, 48

lymphocytes, 60
lymphoma, 61, 62

M

magazines, 43
magnets, 17
majority, 62, 64
malabsorption, 55
malaise, 18
malignancy, 62
maltose, 66
management, 57, 67
matter, 34, 65
meat, 59
medical, 10, 21, 27, 32, 35, 43, 51, 67
medical history, 54
medicine, 64
messages, 43
Mexico, 17
molecules, 60
mortality, 62
mortality rate, 62
motels, 17
motivation, 63
mucosa, 55, 58, 60, 62
muscles, 7, 14, 27, 64
music, 43
mutation, 34

N

National Health and Nutrition Examination Survey, 66
nausea, 9, 39, 63
nerve, 55
neurons, 2
Nile, 33
nurses, 15, 23, 25, 27, 68
nutrition, 34

O

oesophagus, 55

orbit, 21
organs, 56
originality, 11
outpatient, 64

P

pain, 24, 36, 40, 51, 53
paints, 36
palpitations, 63
parallel, 33
parents, 60
pasta, 19, 33, 34, 40, 56, 58, 59
pathologist, 33, 55
pathophysiology, 54
perforation, 29
personal life, 63
persuasion, 31
physicians, 68
plaque, 4
playing, 29, 44
poison, 49
population, 53, 57, 60, 62
problem-solving strategies, 64
professional relationships, 68
proteins, 56, 60
psychiatrist, 64
psychologist, 9, 13, 25, 64, 67

Q

quality of life, 53, 56, 60, 61, 67
questioning, 18

R

rancid, 14
reactions, 32
reading, 13, 43, 48, 59
reality, vii, 40, 41
recovery, 62
relatives, 17, 60
relaxation, 32
remission, 65

response, 65
restaurants, 49, 59
rings, 31, 36
risk, 55, 60, 62
roots, 33

S

sacrum, 48
sadness, 64
safety, 40
scent, 17, 36
school, 39
self-confidence, 14, 15
seminars, 9, 10
sensation, 39
sensations, 32, 39, 53
sensitivity, 20, 65, 66
serology, 62
sex, 15
shape, 7, 17
showing, 36, 44, 58
siblings, 32
signs, 9, 39
silk, 13
silver, 11, 43
skin, 7, 29, 44
smog, 35
social life, 59
social workers, 68
society, 15
solidarity, 21
solitude, 2
solution, 25
spelling, 47
spending, 3, 10, 19
stability, 15
stars, 14, 48
stomach, 27, 28, 33, 55
stress, 18, 29, 68
stretching, 16
stroke, 10
susceptibility, 59
sweeteners, 15

symptoms, 10, 19, 20, 24, 29, 35, 36, 51, 53, 54, 55, 56, 57, 58, 60, 61, 63, 64, 65, 66, 67
syndrome, 2, 26, 53, 54, 61, 68

T

T cell, 62
teachers, 10
techniques, 31
temperature, 54
testing, 18, 57
theatre, 13, 21, 33
therapy, 23, 39
thoughts, vii, 1, 3, 7, 10, 14, 15, 16, 20, 21, 39
tissue, 58
training, 2, 44
trait anxiety, 64
transformation, 27
transfusion, 24
translation, ix
transmission, 64
trauma, 13
treatment, 54, 58, 64, 67
trial, 32
triggers, 56
turtle, 5
twins, 60

U

ulcer, 29, 33

V

vagus nerve, 55
vasovagal syncope, 54
vegetables, 20, 25, 54, 59, 66
velvet, 55
viruses, 3, 34
voting, 44

W

waking, 39
walking, 8, 37, 41
war, 14
water, 10, 22, 33
weakness, 64
wear, 4, 8, 11, 27
web, 25, 49

windows, 14, 17
withdrawal, 58
working conditions, 68
worry, 5, 63

Y

young adults, 53, 56
young people, 34